92 Homeopathic Juice and Meal Recipes to Lower High Blood Pressure:

The Solution to Hypertension Problems without Recurring to Pills or Medicine

By

Joe Correa CSN

COPYRIGHT

© 2017 Live Stronger Faster Inc.

All rights reserved

Reproduction or translation of any part of this work beyond that permitted by section 107 or 108 of the 1976 United States Copyright Act without the permission of the copyright owner is unlawful.

This publication is designed to provide accurate and authoritative information in regard to the subject matter covered. It is sold with the understanding that neither the author nor the publisher is engaged in rendering medical advice. If medical advice or assistance is needed, consult with a doctor. This book is considered a guide and should not be used in any way detrimental to your health. Consult with a physician before starting this nutritional plan to make sure it's right for you.

ACKNOWLEDGEMENTS

This book is dedicated to my friends and family that have had mild or serious illnesses so that you may find a solution and make the necessary changes in your life.

92 Homeopathic Juice and Meal Recipes to Lower High Blood Pressure:

The Solution to Hypertension Problems without Recurring to Pills or Medicine

By

Joe Correa CSN

CONTENTS

ABOUT THE AUTHOR

After years of Research, I honestly believe in the positive effects that proper nutrition can have over the body and mind. My knowledge and experience has helped me live healthier throughout the years and which I have shared with family and friends. The more you know about eating and drinking healthier, the sooner you will want to change your life and eating habits.

Nutrition is a key part in the process of being healthy and living longer so get started today. The first step is the most important and the most significant.

INTRODUCTION

92 Homeopathic Juice and Meal Recipes to Lower High Blood Pressure: The Solution to Hypertension Problems without Recurring to Pills or Medicine

By Joe Correa CSN

Having high blood pressure is becoming more common due to unhealthy eating habits and undue stress. Reducing stress and learning to eat healthier will dramatically reduce your blood pressure.

These juice and meal recipes will help you to quickly and naturally lower your blood pressure in a matter of days. High blood pressure is a serious health condition we all have to face sooner or later. Some people have the tendency to develop it earlier and others once they pass the age of 50.

We have included juices with fruit combinations that include: strawberries, blueberries, lemons, and many more because of their high vitamin C concentration and their powerful effects on dilating blood vessels. We also included juices with watermelon, linseed, bananas, and others because of their high levels of potassium which is an essential element when trying to control hypertension.

Some of the juice and meal recipes have celery and parsley for their phytochemicals and their capacity to eliminate toxins from your body and help control high blood pressure levels.

Try all of these recipes so that you can find the ones you enjoy the most and make them your favorite breakfast, lunch, and dinner options so that you can see you blood pressure normalize again.

92 HOMEOPATHIC JUICE AND MEAL RECIPES TO LOWER HIGH BLOOD PRESSURE: THE SOLUTION TO HYPERTENSION PROBLEMS WITHOUT RECURRING TO PILLS OR MEDICINE

JUICES

1. Avocado and mango juice (2 people)

Ingredients:

- 1 cup of mango cut in slices
- 1/2 cup of avocado cut in cubes
- 2 spoons of honey
- 1/2 cup of natural yogurt
- 1/2 cup of green tea

Procedure: Put the fruits into the fridge for 10 minutes. Mix everything in a blender until you get a creamy look. Add water progressively if you want a more liquid mixture. Serve immediately.

Nutritional facts: Energy 243 kcal, total fat 3 g, cholesterol 7 mg, carbohydrates 69 g and fiber 10 g.

2. Aloe Vera and papaya juice (2 people)

Ingredients:

- 1 aloe Vera leaf
- 1 cup of papaya cut in cubes
- 2 spoons of honey
- 1/2 cup of water
- 1/2 cup of ice cubes

Procedure: Cut the base, lower part and peak of the aloe Vera leaf. Let rest in water what is left for 48 hours. Then open cutting the skin in the middle and with a spoon take all what's inside. We will call this aloe Vera pulp. In a blender mix the papaya, a quarter of cup of the aloe Vera pulp, honey as you like, water and ice.

Nutritional facts: Energy 142 kcal, total fat 0 g, cholesterol 0 mg, carbohydrates 34 g and fiber 2 g.

3. Camu Camu shake (6 people)

Ingredients:

- 3 spoons of camu camu powder or 1 cup of camu camu cut in cubes
- 1 cup of water
- 2 cups of papaya cut in cubes
- 2 cups of strawberries
- 1/2 cup of ice in cubes
- 2 spoons of natural honey

Procedure: In a blender mix the camu camu, strawberries and the ice. Add the honey and mix. Serve in 4 glasses. You can join this powerful shake with oat pancakes

Nutritional facts: Energy 100 kcal, total fat 0 g, cholesterol 0 mg, carbohydrates 22 g and fiber 3 g.

4. Fenugreek smoothie (2 people)

Ingredients:

- 1/4 cup of fenugreek seeds powder
- 1 cup of papaya cut in cubes
- 1/2 cup of green tee
- 1/2 cup of lactose free milk
- 2 spoons of sesame seeds
- 2 spoons of honey

Procedure: Mix everything in a blender until you get a creamy look. Add water progressively if you want a more liquid mixture. Serve in large glasses.

Nutritional facts: Energy 245 kcal, total fat 0 g, cholesterol 0 mg, carbohydrates 46 g and fiber 8 g.

5. Tropical melon shake (4 people)

Ingredients:

- 3 cups of papaya cut in cubes
- 1 cup of mango cut in cubes
- 1 cup of watermelon cut in cubes
- 2 cups of natural yogurt
- 1 ½ cups of pineapple cut in cubes
- 1 cup of ice cubes
- 2 spoons of linseed powder

Procedure: In a blender mix all the ingredients until you get a creamy look. In case you may need something to dissolve if the juice is too dense you can use half cup of water. Serve in long glasses.

Nutritional facts: Energy 194 kcal, total fat 4 g, cholesterol 7 mg, carbohydrates 35 g and fiber 5 g.

6. Non-toxins juice (4 people)

Ingredients:

- 6 strawberries cut in cubes
- 4 chopped plums
- 2 almonds
- juice from ½ lemon
- 2 spoons of raw beetroot
- 2 spoons of grated carrots
- 1 apple cut in cubes without skin
- 1 cup of green tee

Procedure: In a blender mix all the ingredients until you get a creamy look. In case you may need something to dissolve if the juice is too dense you can use half cup of water. Serve in long glasses.

Nutritional facts: Energy 162 kcal, total fat 3 g, cholesterol 8 mg, carbohydrates 64 g and fiber 2 g.

7. Mango and coconut (3 people)

Ingredients:

- 2 cups of coconut juice
- 1 ½ cup of mango cut in cubes

Procedure: You can get coconut juice by cutting a coconut on the top until you break the shell. In case you have no access to fresh coconut you can also use coconut essence by mixing 20 ml of it with 2 cups of water. In a blender mix the coconut juice and the mango. Avoid using honey because the mango has its own natural sweetener. Serve in 2 tall glasses.

Nutritional facts: Energy 149 kcal, total fat 1 g, cholesterol 0 mg, carbohydrates 35 g and fiber 3 g.

8. Strawberry and orange shake (4 people)

Ingredients:

- 1 cup of natural yogurt
- 1 banana
- 1 cup of orange juice
- 8 strawberries

Procedure: Take the green part out from the strawberries and wash. In a blender mix all the ingredients until you get a creamy look. Serve in long glasses.

Nutritional facts: Energy 213 kcal, total fat 0 g, cholesterol 0 mg, carbohydrates 38 g and fiber 3 g.

9. Mint shake (3 people)

Ingredients:

- 1/2 banana
- 1/2 cup of strawberries
- 1/2 cup of orange juice
- 2 mints leaves
- 1 cup of green tee

Procedure: In a blender mix all the ingredients until you get a creamy look. In case you may need something to dissolve if the juice is too dense you can use half cup of water. Serve in long glasses.

Nutritional facts: Energy 232 kcal, total fat 10 g, cholesterol 19 mg, carbohydrates 46 g and fiber 4 g.

10. Peach shake (4 people)

Ingredients:

- 2 cups of peach cut in cubes
- 1 cup of natural yogurt
- 1/3 cup of pineapple cut in cubes
- 1/4 cup of water

Procedure: In a blender mix all the ingredients until you get a creamy look. In case you may need something to dissolve if the juice is too dense you can use half cup of water. Serve in long glasses.

Nutritional facts: Energy 206 kcal, total fat 11 g, cholesterol 6 mg, carbohydrates 54 g and fiber 7 g.

11. Fenugreek fantasy (2 people)

Ingredients:

- 2 cups of fenugreek juice
- 1 cup of chopped parsley leaves
- 2 spoons of sesame seeds
- 1 spoon of linseed powder
- 2 spoons of honey

Procedure: The fenugreek juice is the water from boiling the seeds. You should boil 4 cup of seeds in ½ liter of water in order to get the juice. Then mix everything in a blender until you get a creamy look. Add water progressively if you want a more liquid mixture. Serve in large glasses.

Nutritional facts: Energy 222 kcal, total fat 0 g, cholesterol 0 mg, carbohydrates 48 g and fiber 6 g.

12. Coconut - lemon (5 people)

Ingredients:

- 3/4 cup of lemon juice
- 4 spoons of natural honey
- 1 cup of coconut cream
- 6 ice cubes
- 1/2 cup of coconut in slices
- 1 grated lemon

Procedure: In a blender mix 1 liter of water, lemon juice, honey, coconut cream and ice. Serve and decorate with the coconut and the grated lemon.

Nutritional facts: Energy 234 kcal, total fat 9 g, cholesterol 16 mg, carbohydrates 54 g and fiber 4 g.

13. Delicious Mango (4 people)

Ingredients:

- 2 cups of watermelon cut in slices
- 2 bananas cut in slice
- 1 mango cut in cubes
- 1 cup of natural yogurt
- 1 spoons of natural honey
- 1 cup of ice cubes

Procedure: In a blender mix the watermelon, bananas and mango. Add gradually the yogurt until you get a creamy look. In case you may need something to dissolve if the juice is too dense you can use half cup of water. Add the ice cubes and mix again. Serve in long glasses.

Nutritional facts: Energy 256 kcal, total fat 4 g, cholesterol 8 mg, carbohydrates 68 g and fiber 4 g.

14. Almonds shake (2 people)

Ingredients:

- 1 cup of natural yogurt
- 1 spoon of peanuts (without salt)
- 2 spoons of toasted oats
- 1 spoon of toasted sesame seeds
- 1 spoon of almonds
- 2 spoon of natural honey

Procedure: In a blender pour the glass of almonds milk; add the wheat germ, oats, sesame and almonds. Dress with honey. Serve immediately.

Nutritional facts: Energy 259 kcal, total fat 9 g, cholesterol 14 mg, carbohydrates 32 g and fiber 7 g.

15. Cranberry juice (1 people)

Ingredients:

- 1 cup of organic cranberry juice (250 ml)
- 1/2 cup of water
- 1 spoon of olive oil
- 2 spoons of natural honey

Procedure: Take all the ingredients to the blender and mix until you get a creamy look. It's recommendable to take it every day before breakfast.

Nutritional facts: Energy 198 kcal, total fat 1 g, cholesterol 1 mg, carbohydrates 43 g and fiber 4 g.

16. Watermelon juice (2 people)

Ingredients:

- 4 cups of fresh watermelon
- 3 spoons of fresh parsley leaves
- 1 spoon of natural honey

Procedure: Chop the parsley leaves. Put the watermelon in the blender and mix until you have a liquid and fluid look. Add honey to dress. Serve in tall glasses and pour the basil on top.

Nutritional facts: Energy 187 kcal, total fat 0 g, cholesterol 0 mg, carbohydrates 46 g and fiber 5 g.

17. Parsley juice (2 people)

Ingredients:

- 1 cup of fresh parsley
- 1 green apple
- juice of ½ lemon
- 1/2 spoon of grated ginger
- 1 cup of water

Procedure: Chop the parsley and apple. Introduce all the ingredients to the blender and mix. Strain the juice. Serve in large glasses. Drink before breakfast

Nutritional facts: Energy 222 kcal, total fat 4 g, cholesterol 0 mg, carbohydrates 57 g and fiber 5 g.

18. Lemon juice (2 people)

Ingredients:

- 8 lemons
- 2 glasses of water
- 2 spoons of apple vinegar (30 ml)

Procedure: Squeeze the juice from the lemons and mix with the water and vinegar. To clean your body and kidneys take the juice during mornings at least during a week.

Nutritional facts: Energy 159 kcal, total fat 0 g, cholesterol 0 mg, carbohydrates 32 g and fiber 2 g.

19. Fenugreek milkshake (2 people)

Ingredients:

- 1 cup of fenugreek juice
- 1 cup of almond lactose free milk
- 1/4 cup of chopped almonds
- 2 raisins cut in slices
- 2 spoons of honey

Procedure: Mix everything in a blender until you get a creamy look. Add water progressively if you want a more liquid mixture. Serve in large glasses.

Nutritional facts: Energy 228 kcal, total fat 9 g, cholesterol 28 mg, carbohydrates 46 g and fiber 7 g.

20. Celery and apple juice (2 people)

Ingredients:

- 2 celery steam including the leaves
- 3 apples
- 1 spoon of fresh mint
- 2 spoons of honey
- 1/2 cup of water

Procedure: Cut the celery, apples and mint. Put everything in a blender and mix until you get a creamy look. If you want it more liquid, then you should add water progressively until you get the look you are looking for. Strain the juice and serve.

Nutritional facts: Energy 215 kcal, total fat 0 g, cholesterol 0 mg, carbohydrates 58 g and fiber 3 g.

21. Carrots and celery juice (1 people)

Ingredients:

- 3 big carrots
- 3 celery steams
- 1 cup of water

Procedure: Wash the carrots and the celery. Peel the carrots and then cut in slices. Chop the celery. Put the ingredients in the blender and mix. Serve in tall glasses.

Nutritional facts: Energy 154 kcal, total fat 0 g, cholesterol 0 mg, carbohydrates 27 g and fiber 4 g.

22. Cucumber and parsley juice (2 people)

Ingredients:

- 1/2 cucumber
- 100 gr of parsley
- 1 cup of water

Procedure: Wash the cucumber and parsley. Cut the cucumber in slices and chop the parsley. Put everything in the blender and mix. Strain and serve.

Nutritional facts: Energy 176 kcal, total fat 0 g, cholesterol 0 mg, carbohydrates 35 g and fiber 2 g.

23. Grape juice (2 people)

Ingredients:

- 250 g of red grapes
- 1 cup of water
- 1/2 spoon of mint
- 2 spoons of honey

Procedure: Wash the grapes. Peel the grapes and then cut by the half to take the seeds out. Put everything in a blender and mix. Serve immediately.

Nutritional facts: Energy 165 kcal, total fat 0 g, cholesterol 0 mg, carbohydrates 36 g and fiber 4 g.

24. Watermelon and lemon juice (2 people)

Ingredients:

- 4 cups of fresh watermelon cut in cubes
- 4 spoons of lemon juice
- 1/2 cup of water
- 2 spoons of honey

Procedure: Mix everything in a blender until you get a creamy look. Dress with honey and mix again. Serve in tall glasses.

Nutritional facts: Energy 175 kcal, total fat 0 g, cholesterol 0 mg, carbohydrates 28 g and fiber 3 g.

25. Watermelon and celery juice (2 people)

Ingredients:

- 3 cups of watermelon
- 3 celery steams
- 2 spoons of natural honey
- 1 cup of water

Procedure: Wash the celery. Peel the watermelon and cut in thin slices. Chop the celery. Join together with the water in a blender and mix. Strain and serve in tall glasses.

Nutritional facts: Energy 176 kcal, total fat 0 g, cholesterol 0 mg, carbohydrates 31 g and fiber 2 g.

26. Body cleaner juice (2 people)

Ingredients:

- 1/2 cabbage
- 1 carrot
- 2 celery steams
- 1/2 cup of germinated beans
- 1 cup of pineapple
- 1 cup of water

Procedure: Mix everything in a blender and add water progressively. Once you have a creamy look you are ready to strain the juice. Serve and enjoy.

Nutritional facts: Energy 232 kcal, total fat 2 g, cholesterol 2 mg, carbohydrates 47 g and fiber 6 g.

27. Acai-berry mix juice (2 people)

Ingredients:

- 1/2 cup of orange juice
- 1 banana cut in slices
- 1 mango cut in slices
- 1 cup of pulp of acai berries
- 1 cup of water
- 2 spoons of natural honey

Procedure: Mix everything in a blender and add water progressively according to the consistence you want to get. Once you have a creamy look serve and enjoy.

Nutritional facts: Energy 276 kcal, total fat 10 g, cholesterol 9 mg, carbohydrates 64 g and fiber 5 g.

28. Blood pressure special juice (2 people)

Ingredients:

- 4 carrots
- 2 apples
- 1 piece of ginger (5 cm)
- 1/2 cup of coconut juice
- 1 cup of water

Procedure: Wash all the ingredients. Peel the carrots and ginger. Chop the carrots and apples. Mix everything in a blender. Serve immediately.

Nutritional facts: Energy 245 kcal, total fat 4 g, cholesterol 7 mg, carbohydrates 43 g and fiber 4 g.

29. Fenugreek and papaya juice (2 people)

Ingredients:

- 1 cup of fenugreek juice
- 1 cup of papaya cut in cubes
- 1 cup of green tee
- 2 spoons of sesame seeds
- 2 spoons of honey

Procedure: Consider that the fenugreek juice is obtained by boiling the seeds in a pot with ½ liter of water. The water you get from it is the juice, you can reserve the rest for the next days and mix it with your juices. Now mix everything in a blender until you get a creamy look. Add water progressively if you want a more liquid mixture. Serve immediately.

Nutritional facts: Energy 245 kcal, total fat 3 g, cholesterol 8 mg, carbohydrates 76 g and fiber 8 g.

30. Pumpkin juice (2 people)

Ingredients:

- 1 glass of water
- 1 glass of coconut juice
- 1/2 cup of cooked pumpkin
- 1 spoon of honey

Procedure: In a blender mix the coconut, water and pumpkin for some minutes until you get a creamy look. Pour the juice in tall glasses and add the honey and mix again. Enjoy.

Nutritional facts: Energy 198 kcal, total fat 2 g, cholesterol 6 mg, carbohydrates 66 g and fiber 4 g.

31. Blueberry juice (2 people)

Ingredients:

- 1 cup of natural yogurt
- 1 cup of blueberries
- 1 spoon of linseed powder
- 1/4 cup of water

Procedure: Wash the blueberries. Mix everything in a blender until you get a creamy look. Add water progressively if you want a more liquid mixture. Serve immediately.

Nutritional facts: Energy 198 kcal, total fat 11 g, cholesterol 21 mg, carbohydrates 54 g and fiber 2 g.

32. Orange shake (2 people)

Ingredients:

- 1 cup of orange juice
- 1/2 cup of water
- 1/2 spoon of vanilla essence
- 2 spoons of honey
- 1/2 cup of natural yogurt
- 5 ice cubes

Procedure: Mix everything in a blender until you get a creamy look. Add water progressively if you want a more liquid mixture. Serve immediately.

Nutritional facts: Energy 212 kcal, total fat 3 g, cholesterol 6 mg, carbohydrates 48 g and fiber 2 g.

33. Apple-carrot juice (2 people)

Ingredients:

- 2 cups of orange juice
- 1 cut of chop apple
- 6 carrots cut in cubes
- 2 spoons of honey

Procedure: Mix everything in a blender until you get a creamy look. Add water progressively if you want a more liquid mixture. Serve immediately.

Nutritional facts: Energy 198 kcal, total fat 5 g, cholesterol 2 mg, carbohydrates 62 g and fiber 5 g.

34. Super banana booster (2 people)

Ingredients:

- 3/4 cup of milk
- 1/4 cup of granola
- 1 banana
- 1 cup of ice cubes
- 2 spoons of linseed powder

Procedure: Mix everything in a blender until you get a creamy look. Add water progressively if you want a more liquid mixture. Serve in tall glasses.

Nutritional facts: Energy 276 kcal, total fat 7 g, cholesterol 7 mg, carbohydrates 32 g and fiber 7 g.

35. Spinach banana (2 people)

Ingredients:

- 1 banana
- 1/2 cup of chopped spinach
- 1 spoon of peanut butter
- 1 ½ cup of lactose free milk
- 1 spoon of linseed powder
- 1 spoon of sesame seeds

Procedure: Mix everything in a blender until you get a creamy look. Add water progressively if you want a more liquid mixture. Serve in tall glasses. Decorate with sesame seeds and enjoy.

Nutritional facts: Energy 230 kcal, total fat 9 g, cholesterol 9 mg, carbohydrates 23 g and fiber 7 g.

36. Kale power juice (2 people)

Ingredients:

- 1 cup of fresh kale
- 1 cup of almond milk
- 1 cup of blueberries
- 1/2 banana
- 1 spoon of almond butter
- 2 spoon of instant oats

Procedure: Mix everything in a blender until you get a creamy look. Add water progressively if you want a more liquid mixture. Serve immediately.

Nutritional facts: Energy 256 kcal, total fat 9 g, cholesterol 8 mg, carbohydrates 25 g and fiber 12 g.

37. Blueberry-oats juice (2 people)

Ingredients:

- 1 banana
- 1 cup of blueberries
- 1/3 cup of instant oats
- 1 cup of lactose free milk

Procedure: Put the banana and blueberries in the fridge for 10 minutes. Mix everything in a blender until you get a creamy look. Add water progressively if you want a more liquid mixture. Serve in tall glasses.

Nutritional facts: Energy 214 kcal, total fat 4 g, cholesterol 0 mg, carbohydrates 64 g and fiber 4 g.

38. Red delights (2 people)

Ingredients:

- 1/2 cup of raspberries
- 1 cup of strawberries
- 1 cup of mango
- 1 cup of water
- 2 spoons of honey

Procedure: Put the fruits into the fridge for 10 minutes. Mix everything in a blender until you get a creamy look. Add water progressively if you want a more liquid mixture. Serve immediately.

Nutritional facts: Energy 214 kcal, total fat 5 g, cholesterol 0 mg, carbohydrates 48 g and fiber 4 g.

39. Blue delights (2 people)

Ingredients:

- 1 cup of raspberries
- 1 cup of blueberries
- 1 cup of strawberries
- 1/2 cup of natural yogurt
- 1/2 cup of green tee

Procedure: Mix everything in a blender until you get a creamy look. Add the water progressively if you want a more liquid mixture. Serve in tall glasses.

Nutritional facts: Energy 198 kcal, total fat 4 g, cholesterol 5 mg, carbohydrates 38 g and fiber 4 g.

40. Straw-nana juice (2 people)

Ingredients:

- 1/2 cup of chopped pineapple
- 1 banana
- 1/2 cup of mango cut in slices
- 1 cup of strawberries
- 1 cup of lactose free milk

Procedure: Mix everything in a blender until you get a creamy look. Add water progressively if you want a more liquid mixture. Serve immediately.

Nutritional facts: Energy 215 kcal, total fat 3 g, cholesterol 6 mg, carbohydrates 53 g and fiber 5 g.

41. Green delights (2 people)

Ingredients:

- 1 chopped kiwi
- 1 ½ cups of watermelon cut in cubes
- 1 ½ cups of red grapes
- 1 cup of lactose free milk
- 1 spoon of vanilla essence
- 1 spoon of honey

Procedure: Peel the grapes and then cut by the half. Take all the seeds out and chop. Mix everything in a blender until you get a creamy look. Add water progressively if you want a more liquid mixture. Serve immediately.

Nutritional facts: Energy 245 kcal, total fat 6 g, cholesterol 7 mg, carbohydrates 48 g and fiber 5 g.

42. Mango delights (2 people)

Ingredients:

- 2 mangos cut in slices
- 1 cup of natural yogurt
- 1 cup of water
- 1 banana
- 2 spoons of lemon juice
- 1 spoon of vanilla essence

Procedure: Mix everything in a blender until you get a creamy look. Add water progressively if you want a more liquid mixture. Serve in large glasses.

Nutritional facts: Energy 198 kcal, total fat 3 g, cholesterol 7 mg, carbohydrates 46 g and fiber 4 g.

43. Apple and lemon juice (2 people)

Ingredients:

- 2 green apples cut in cubes
- -6 leaves of kale
- 2 steams of celery
- 1/2 spoon of lemon juice
- 1 cucumber

Procedure: Wash and chop the kale, cucumber and celery. Mix everything in a blender until you get a creamy look. Add water progressively if you want a more liquid mixture. Serve in large glasses.

Nutritional facts: Energy 187 kcal, total fat 3 g, cholesterol 0 mg, carbohydrates 56 g and fiber 4 g.

44. Raspberry-mint delight (2 people)

Ingredients:

- 2 cups of raspberries cut in cubes
- 1 cup of water
- 3/4 of natural yogurt
- 1 cup of chopped mango
- 1/2 cup of chopped mint leaves
- 1 spoon of lemon juice
- 1 pinch of salt
- 1/2 cup of ice cubes

Procedure: Take the fruits to the fridge for 10 minutes. Mix everything in a blender until you get a creamy look. Add water progressively if you want a more liquid mixture. Serve immediately.

Nutritional facts: Energy 243 kcal, total fat 3 g, cholesterol 7 mg, carbohydrates 54 g and fiber 7 g.

MEALS

1. Oat bran muffins with raisins and walnuts

Benefits: Using high in fiber oat bran as flour substitution makes this recipe especially suitable to lower blood pressure and improve digestive health. Raisins, provided they are made from organic grapes, are not only rich in potassium but also provide a rich sweet flavor in this healthy breakfast option.

Ingredients:

- 180 g oat bran
- 30 ml low fat milk
- 1 egg
- 4 tbsp. honey
- 2 tbsp. coconut oil (optional)
- 0,5 tsp baking powder
- 30 g raisins
- 30 g walnuts

How to prepare:

Whisk together an egg, honey, milk and melted coconut oil. Incorporate oat bran and baking powder. Pour the mixture into individual paper muffin baking cups. Bake for 15 minutes at 425 F until golden brown. Makes 7 muffins.

Per serving: 182 calories, sodium 116 mg, potassium 114 mg, sugars 7 g

2. Oat bran banana pancakes

Benefits: Banana and oat bran are both amazing sources of potassium. Banana and low-fat yogurt are the base of these delicious breakfast pancakes and will help you to lose weight, lower your blood pressure, and boost energy levels throughout the day.

Ingredients:

- 100 g oat bran
- 1 ripe banana
- 80 g plain low fat yogurt
- 2 tbsp. honey
- baking powder

How to prepare: Mash the banana and combine it with low fat yogurt and honey, incorporate oat bran and baking powder. Pour about 2 tablespoons per pancake onto a pan and fry in coconut or olive oil until crispy on both sides. Makes about 8 pancakes.

Per serving: 66 calories, sodium 58 mg, potassium 97 mg, sugars 6 g

3. Warm oatmeal with prunes and mixed nuts

Benefits: Prunes have always been considered one of the best digestive remedies. They are also a good source of potassium and have a variety of minerals. Nuts are packed with protein, fiber and essential fats.

Ingredients:

- 100 g oats
- 150 ml low fat milk
- 50 g diced dried prunes
- 40 g chopped walnuts, pistachios, hazelnuts etc.

How to prepare: Bring milk to a simmer in a saucepan, add diced prunes and oats, simmer for 8 minutes on low heat while stirring. Top with cinnamon and chopped nuts. Makes 3 servings.

Per serving: 270 calories, sodium 25 mg, potassium 390 mg, sugars 9 g

4. "Baklava" diet breakfast

Benefits: Tangerines are packed with flavonoids, vitamin C, vitamin A, folate, and potassium. Low fat yogurt is an awesome source of calcium, vitamin B- 2, vitamin B- 12, potassium, and magnesium.

Ingredients:

- 150 g low fat Greek yogurt
- 1 tbsp. honey
- 20 g pistachios
- 10 g almonds
- 1 small tangerine

How to prepare: Chop pistachios and almonds, add diced tangerine. Pour Greek yogurt and honey over the mixture and mix thoroughly. Makes 2 servings.

Per serving: 114 calories, sodium 162 mg, potassium 157 mg, sugars 5 g

5. Oatmeal with pecans, plums and honey

Benefits: Pecans are high in healthy unsaturated fat and contain more than 19 vitamins and minerals including vitamins A, B, and E, folic acid, calcium, magnesium, phosphorus, potassium, and zinc. Plums will satisfy your hunger for a very long time.

Ingredients:

- 100 g oats
- 150 ml low fat milk
- 20 g chopped pecans
- 2 plums
- 2 tbsp. honey

How to prepare: Bring milk to a simmer in a saucepan, add oats simmer for 8 minutes on low heat while stirring. Top with chopped pecans and diced plums. Finish with a drizzle of honey. Makes 3 servings.

Per serving: 230 calories, sodium 25 mg, potassium 233 mg, sugars 9 g

6. Exotic raw buckwheat breakfast porridge

Benefits: Buckwheat is a super-food that is excellent for digestion and blood pressure. It is one of the best sources of high-quality, easily digestible protein. Kiwis are considered one of the best fruits to lower your blood pressure.

Ingredients:

- 200 g raw buckwheat
- 200 ml water
- 150 ml low fat milk
- 1 kiwi
- 30 g melon

How to prepare: Leave buckwheat covered in water overnight. Drain the water and put buckwheat, milk, diced kiwi and melon to a blender and mix well. Makes 4 servings.

Per serving: 220 calories, sodium 23 mg, potassium 319 mg, sugars 3.5 g

7. Summer berries yogurt bowl

Benefits: Strawberries, blueberries and raspberries are rich in nutrients, antioxidants and phytochemicals which may help prevent and reverse diabetes, high blood pressure and, even certain types of cancer.

Ingredients:

- 200 g low fat yogurt
- 50 g fresh blueberries
- 50 g fresh strawberries
- 50 g fresh raspberries
- 50 g oats

How to prepare: Combine berries, yogurt and oats together in a bowl and serve. Makes 3 servings.

Per serving: 90 calories, sodium 48 mg, potassium 280 mg, sugars 7 g

8. Plum and nectarine smoothie

Benefits: Nectarines are very rich in beta-carotene, vitamin A, vitamin C, fiber and potassium. Plums contain no saturated fats and are full of minerals and vitamins.

Ingredients:

- 100 g low fat yogurt
- 150 ml low fat milk
- 4 medium ripe plums
- 1 nectarine

How to prepare: Put yogurt, milk, diced peeled plums and nectarine and mix well. Pour into glasses and serve. Makes 2 servings.

Per serving: 99 calories, sodium 69 mg, potassium 376 mg, sugars 12 g

9. Creamy buckwheat

Benefits: This recipe possesses all the benefits of super-foods like buckwheat and banana. Low fat milk makes it especially diet-friendly and healthy.

Ingredients:

- 100 g buckwheat
- 200 ml water
- 40 ml low fat milk
- 1 banana
- 2 tbsp. honey

How to prepare: Bring water to a boil in a saucepan, add buckwheat and simmer for 10 minutes or until it soaks all the liquid. Add diced bananas and drizzle with honey. Makes 4 servings.

Per serving: 157 calories, sodium 20 mg, potassium 218 mg, sugars 9 g

10. Baked apples with oats and nuts

Benefits: Apples are extremely rich in important antioxidants, flavonoids, and dietary fiber, they may help reduce the risk of developing cancer, hypertension, diabetes, and heart disease.

Ingredients:

- 2 medium apples
- 3 tbsp. honey
- 40 g oats
- 30 g walnuts or pecans

How to prepare: Peel apples and cut them in half, remove the hull and place apples onto a baking tray lined with parchment paper. Chop walnuts or pecans, mix them with oats and top apples with the mixture. Drizzle honey on top and place in a preheated oven at 370 degrees F for 20 minutes or until apples are tender and golden. Makes 4 servings.

Per serving: 179 calories, sodium 2 mg, potassium 181 mg, sugars 4 g

11. Breakfast quinoa salad with baked peaches and nuts

Benefits: Quinoa contains iron, magnesium, potassium, calcium, vitamin E, and fiber. Peaches offer a rich variety of calcium, potassium, magnesium.

Ingredients:

- 50 g quinoa
- 150 ml water
- 40 ml low fat milk
- 2 medium peaches
- 40 g pistachios

How to prepare: Chop the peaches, place them onto a cooking tray, drizzle with honey and bake at 400 degrees F for about 25 minutes. Meanwhile cook your quinoa as stated on the packaging. Combine chopped pistachios, peaches and quinoa, pour in room temperature milk and serve warm. Makes 3 servings.

Per serving: 164 calories, sodium 80 mg, potassium 377 mg, sugars 6 g

12. Light panna cotta with apricots honey and walnuts

Benefits: This low fat creamy and delicate dessert may become one of your favorites. Apricots provide you with fiber, potassium, iron, and antioxidants.

Ingredients:

- 200 g low fat yogurt
- 100 ml low fat milk
- vanilla extract
- gelatin or agar
- 1 tbsp. honey
- 2 small apricots
- 30 g walnuts

How to prepare: Cover gelatin or agar with water and leave it to soak for 10 minutes, meanwhile heat your milk and yogurt in a saucepan while stirring in order to prevent any lumps. Add 1 tbsp. honey for sweetness. Dice your apricots, combine with chopped walnuts and evenly distribute the mixture between 3 little baking sheets. Incorporate gelatin or agar into the liquid and pour onto the sheets. Leave them in a freezer for at least 6 hours. Sprinkle with chopped walnuts and drizzle with honey (optional). Makes 3 servings.

Per serving: 156 calories, sodium 63 mg, potassium 324 mg, sugars 10 g

13. Blueberries, plum and hazelnut salad

Benefits: This recipe possesses all the benefits of plums and blueberries, as well as hazelnuts. Hazelnuts are rich in unsaturated fats, high in magnesium, calcium and vitamins B and E.

Ingredients:

- 150 g blueberries
- 4 medium plums
- 40 g hazelnuts
- leafy greens of your choice

How to prepare: Dice your plums and chop your hazelnuts. Combine all the ingredients together in a salad bowl and serve. Makes 2 servings.

Per serving: 139 calories, sodium 0 mg, potassium 221 mg, sugars 5 g

14. Baked pumpkin and carrot salad

Benefits: Pumpkin helps you to lower blood pressure and is extremely beneficial for your heart. Carrots are rich in vitamin A, Vitamin C, Vitamin K, vitamin B8, pantothenic acid, folate, potassium, iron, copper, and manganese.

Ingredients:

- 200 g pumpkin
- 100 g carrot
- 100 g feta cheese
- 1 tbsp. honey
- 30 g pine nuts

How to prepare: Dice your pumpkin and carrots, drizzle with honey and bake until tender at 400 degrees F. Cut feta cheese into small cubes. Combine all the ingredients together and serve. Makes 3 servings.

Per serving: 139 calories, sodium 0 mg, potassium 221 mg, sugars 5 g

15. Cherry tomato pomegranate salad

Benefits: Cherry tomatoes are a good source of vitamins and minerals essential for good health. Pomegranates are proven to have blood pressure-reducing properties.

Ingredients:

- 150 g cherry tomatoes
- 1 medium pomegranate
- 1 medium red onion
- 50 g feta cheese

How to prepare: Cut cherry tomatoes in half, roughly chop the onion and feta cheese and combine with the pomegranate. Drizzle with lemon juice (optional) and serve. Makes 3 servings.

Per serving: 101 calories, sodium 190 mg, potassium 316 mg, sugars 10 g

16. Green salad with creamy avocado sauce

Benefits: Broccoli is a very good source of dietary fiber, vitamin B6, vitamin E, manganese, vitamin B1, vitamin A, potassium and calcium. Incredibly nutritious and packed with potassium and other minerals avocado is essential to have in your diet.

Ingredients:

- 100 g broccoli
- 100 g green peas
- spinach (to taste)
- 0.5 ripe avocado
- 50 g low fat yogurt

How to prepare: Boil your broccoli for 15 minutes and chop them. Combine with peas and fresh spinach leaves. Put avocado pulp and yogurt in a blender and mix thoroughly. Pour the sauce on top of the salad and drizzle with lemon juice or olive oil (optional). Makes 2 servings.

Per serving: 184 calories, sodium 59 mg, potassium 722 mg, sugars 5 g

17. Sweet potato patties with spinach and mushrooms

Benefits: Sweet potatoes are an excellent source of vitamin A, vitamin C, manganese, copper, pantothenic acid and potassium. Spinach is packed with protein, fiber, vitamins A, C, E and K, thiamin, vitamin B6, calcium, iron, magnesium, phosphorus, and potassium.

Ingredients:

- 100 g sweet potato
- Spinach
- 100 g mushrooms
- 1 small red onion
- Olive oil
- 60 g buckwheat flour

How to prepare: Chop the onion finely and fry in olive oil until slightly brown. Chop the mushrooms and add to the pan. Fry for 20 minutes on low heat while adding tiny bit of water if needed, add finely chopped spinach leaves and fry for another 5 minutes. Meanwhile boil your sweet potato and mushrooms with little bit of olive oil. Combine mushrooms, mushed sweet potato and buckwheat flour.

Form the patties and fry them in olive oil until ready on both sides. Makes 5 patties.

Per serving: 111 calories, sodium 10 mg, potassium 228 mg, sugars 1 g

18. Corn chowder with white beans and cauliflower

Benefits: Corn is a rich source of many vitamins and minerals. By eating fiber-rich white beans you can reduce the risk of having cancer and high blood pressure.

Ingredients:

- 100 g sweet corn
- 50 g white beans
- 2 small potatoes
- 100 g cauliflower
- 50 ml low fat milk
- 1 medium onion

How to prepare: Peel, roughly chop and boil the potatoes until ready. Add milk and let cool down. Meanwhile fry your chopped onion in olive oil with crumbled cauliflower for about 15 minutes until golden brown. In a saucepan combine the potatoes with liquid, cauliflower, add cooked beans and sweet corn. Serve warm. Add a little bit of low fat cheese on top (optional). Makes 3 servings.

Per serving: 191 calories, sodium 29 mg, potassium 1018 mg, sugars 5.9 g

19. Grilled watermelon with pomegranate, feta cheese and orange

Benefits: Watermelon is a significant source of vitamins A, B6 and C, antioxidants, amino acids and potassium. Feta cheese supplies key vitamins and minerals for your diet.

Ingredients:

- 100 g watermelon
- 70 g feta cheese
- 1 medium pomegranate
- 0.5 medium orange

How to prepare: Chop your watermelon (don't forget to take away the seeds), place it onto the cooking tray and set your oven to grill mode (alternatively use a normal grill oven), cook the watermelon until it is slightly tender on the sides. Cut feta cheese into cubes and combine with diced orange and pomegranate. Add grilled watermelon and serve as soon as possible. Makes 2 servings.

Per serving: 157 calories, sodium 391 mg, potassium 277 mg, sugars 15 g

20. Russian diet cabbage soup

Benefits: Potatoes are very high in potassium and if eaten in moderation will only have positive impact on your health. This soup is extremely low fat and will help you lose all those extra pounds and boost your metabolism.

Ingredients:

- 100 g cabbage
- 100 g carrots
- 1 medium onion
- 2 small potatoes
- parsley and dill (to taste)

How to prepare: Combine grated carrots and chopped onion together on a frying pan and fry for 10 minutes until golden brown. Meanwhile cut the cabbage and potatoes into medium pieces of same size and start boiling them. Halfway through (after about 15 minutes) add the carrots and leave the soup to simmer on medium heat for another 15- 20 minutes. Add chopped parsley and dill. Makes 3 servings.

Per serving: 101 calories, sodium 14 mg, potassium 571 mg, sugars 4 g

21. Sweet potato carrot pumpkin soup with cumin and coriander

Benefits: This soup is packed with potassium and other blood pressure lowering minerals.

Ingredients:

- 1 medium sweet potato
- 2 carrots
- 100 g pumpkin
- 1 medium red onion
- 100 ml low fat milk (preferably almond milk)
- cumin (to taste)
- coriander (to taste)

How to prepare: Shred sweet potato, carrots and pumpkin into a bowl and mix well. In a saucepan heat 1 tbsp. of olive oil and fry the chopped onion until tender. Add a little bit of olive oil and combine with the shredded vegetables, all cumin and coriander to taste and mix well. Pour milk into the saucepan slowly while stirring and leave on a low heat for 30 minutes. Turn off the heat and let cool. Using blender create a smooth creamy consistency. Serve warm, add pumpkin seeds or shredded coconut on top (optional). Makes 2 servings.

Per serving: 197 calories, sodium 90 mg, potassium 726 mg, sugars 12 g

22. Cauliflower crust pumpkin pizza

Benefits: Cauliflower is a good source of vitamin C, protein, thiamin, riboflavin, niacin, magnesium, phosphorus, fiber, vitamin B6, folate, pantothenic acid, potassium, and manganese. Enjoy your pizza without having to worry about gaining weight.

Ingredients:

- 100 g cauliflower
- 1 large red onions
- 50 g pumpkin
- 50 g tomato puree
- basil (to taste)
- 40 g buckwheat flour
- 1 small egg
- 40 g low fat cheese or mozzarella

How to prepare: Boil cauliflower for 5 minutes on medium heat and put in a blender. Drain well and spread on a towel until it dries. Beat one egg and combine with the cauliflower and buckwheat flour, knead for a while and spread on parchment paper. Cook the sauce: mix shredded pumpkin with pureed tomatoes and chopped onion and simmer for 15 minutes until relatively thick. Add basil (optional). Spread sauce over the crust, add shredded low fat cheese or mozzarella on top and bake for 30 minutes at 425 degrees F.

Per whole pizza: 377 calories, sodium 354 mg, potassium 1151 mg, sugars 14 g

23. Light beet and orange salad

Benefits: Beets are high in immune-boosting vitamin C, fiber, and essential minerals like potassium and manganese. Oranges are an excellent source of vitamin C, dietary fiber, vitamin A, calcium, copper, and potassium.

Ingredients:

- 1 medium beet
- 1 medium orange
- 40 g pine nuts
- spinach
- 30 g low fat yogurt

How to prepare: Boil the beets and cut into cubes, dice the oranges. Mix all the ingredients together. Drizzle with yogurt and serve. Makes 3 servings.

Per serving: 143 calories, sodium 43 mg, potassium 390 mg, sugars 8 g

24. Mashed potatoes with light mushrooms sauce

Benefits: Mushrooms are also a good source of selenium, an antioxidant mineral, as well as copper, niacin, potassium and phosphorous. Additionally, mushrooms provide protein, vitamin C and iron. Combined with mashed potatoes they create a classic creamy flavor.

Ingredients:

- 2 medium potatoes
- 100 g mushrooms
- 100g low fat yogurt
- 30 g low fat cheese

How to prepare: Wash the potatoes thoroughly but don't peel. Bake for 30 minutes or until tender at 400 degrees F. Meanwhile roughly chop the mushrooms and fry in olive oil for 20 minutes. Let the potatoes cool, cut in half lengthwise and take away the contents. Mash it up and combine with yogurt and mushrooms. Stuff the potatoes again, put shredded cheese on top and bake for another 5 minutes. Makes 2 servings.

Per serving: 143 calories, sodium 43 mg, potassium 390 mg, sugars 8 g

25. Mushroom and carrot pot pie

Benefits: This recipe is an awesome alternative to the usual pot pie, though it doesn't lack taste and remains to be an awesome example of a comfort food.

Ingredients:

- 100 g mushrooms
- 100g carrots
- 50 g potatoes
- 40 g low fat yogurt
- 30 g low fat cheese
- 1 medium red onion

How to prepare: Combine shredded carrots, chopped mushrooms and onion on a pan and fry them for 20 minutes on low heat while adding water if necessary. Meanwhile boil the potatoes and mash them with yogurt. Put mushrooms to the bottom of a baking sheet, then cover with mashed potatoes and add shredded cheese on top. Bake for 30 minutes at 400 degrees F. Makes 2 servings.

Per serving: 98calories, sodium 113 mg, potassium 511 mg, sugars 6 g

26. Avocado carrot and orange salad with spinach and feta cheese

Benefits: This recipe combines some of the best foods to lower your high blood pressure and is very beneficial for your digestive health and heart.

Ingredients:

- 1 ripe avocado
- 100g carrots
- 100 g orange
- spinach
- 100 g feta cheese
- 1 tbsp. honey

How to prepare: Cut carrots into rings, drizzle with honey and fry in olive oil until slightly golden. Cut avocado, oranges and feta cheese into cubes. Combine all the ingredients and serve. Makes 3 servings.

Per serving: 260 calories, sodium 399 mg, potassium 456 mg, sugars 9 g

27. Stuffed cabbage leaves

Benefits: Black rice, a super-food that is gaining popularity these days and is very beneficial for your immune health. Raisins are a great source of B vitamins, iron, and potassium.

Ingredients:

- 3 medium whole cabbage leaves
- 100 g black rice
- 100 g basmati rice
- 50 g raisins
- curry powder (to taste)
- turmeric (to taste)

How to prepare: Boil cabbage leaves until tender. Meanwhile cook both types of rice according to the packaging in which they came in. Add curry powder and turmeric, combine with the raisins and put the mixture inside each cabbage leaf. Serve warm. Makes 3 servings.

Per serving: 230 calories, sodium 9 mg, potassium 227 mg, sugars 10 g

28. Quinoa primavera

Benefits: A great alternative to a traditional Spanish pasta primavera and is packed with healthy nutrients, low in calories, and high in protein.

Ingredients:

- 100 g quinoa
- 100 g broccoli
- 50 g peas
- 100 g cherry tomatoes
- 1 small carrot

How to prepare: Chop all the vegetables and put into a saucepan. Drizzle with olive oil and fry for 5 minutes. Thoroughly wash quinoa and put into the saucepan. Cover with water and boil until all the liquid is absorbed. Makes 3 servings.

Per serving: 160 calories, sodium 26 mg, potassium 466 mg, sugars 3 g

29. Eggplants baked in tomato sauce

Benefits: Eggplants are an excellent source of dietary fiber, vitamins B1 and B6, potassium, and various minerals. Tomatoes are packed with vitamin C, biotin, molybdenum and vitamin K, copper, potassium, manganese, dietary fiber, vitamin A, vitamin B6, folate, niacin, vitamin E, and phosphorus.

Ingredients:

- 1 medium eggplants
- 2 giant tomatoes
- 1 medium bell pepper
- 50 g olives
- 1 medium red onion
- 50 g mozzarella
- basil (to taste)
- rosemary (to taste)

How to prepare: Finely chop the onion and fry until golden brown, add chopped tomatoes, pepper, olives and spices. Simmer for 15 minutes on medium heat. Meanwhile slice the eggplant and cover with cold salted water. Let it sit until the sauce is ready. Lay eggplant at the bottom of a baking sheet or dish pan and cover with sauce. Put mozzarella on top and bake for 40 minutes at 400 degrees F. Makes 3 servings.

Per serving: 140 calories, sodium 254 mg, potassium 380 mg, sugars 5 g

30. Baked beans

Benefits: Apples, carrots, and tomatoes: three of the best foods for weight loss together. Kidney beans are an awesome source of fiber and are considered one of the best health-promoting foods.

Ingredients:

- 100 g apples
- 100 g carrots
- 1 can of red beans
- 100 g tomato puree
- rosemary (to taste)
- oregano (to taste)

How to prepare: Shred apples and carrots and mix together. Combine the shredded mix, tomato puree and beans. Add rosemary and oregano and bake for 20 minutes at 400 degrees F. Makes 3 servings.

Per serving: 250 calories, sodium 40 mg, potassium 1122 mg, sugars 8 g

31. Curried cauliflower

Benefits: Curry, apart from having a unique flavor that goes with literally any vegetable, is also a great immune health booster. Cauliflower is perfect for weight loss and digestive health improvement.

Ingredients:

- 200 g cauliflower
- curry (to taste)
- 2 tbsp. lemon juice
- coriander (to taste)

How to prepare: Roughly chop or crumble cauliflower, drizzle with olive oil and lemon juice, add curry powder and coriander and bake for 20 minutes at 400 degrees F. Makes 2 servings.

Per serving: 110 calories, sodium 33 mg, potassium 380 mg, sugars 2 g

32. Beans and zucchini patties

Benefits: Zucchini has a high content of vitamin A, **magnesium**, **folate**, **potassium**, copper, and **protein**. Buckwheat flour is a great substitute to wheat flour, it's low in calories and also very beneficial to your health.

Ingredients:

- 1 medium zucchini
- 1 can black beans
- 1 medium red onion
- chili (to taste)
- cumin (to taste)
- 50 g buckwheat flour

How to prepare: Roughly chop the onion and fry in olive oil until golden brown, add chili powder and cumin. Shred zucchini and put in a blender with beans and onion. Blend well, add flour and form patties. Fry on both sides until crispy. Makes 6 patties.

Per serving: 151 calories, sodium 7 mg, potassium 460 mg, sugars 2 g

33. Baked potatoes with polenta and rosemary

Benefits: Polenta is a low carbohydrate food rich in vitamin A and C. It has health benefits such as cancer and heart disease prevention.

Ingredients:

- 4 small potatoes
- 50 g polenta
- rosemary
- 50 g low fat yogurt

How to prepare: Wash potatoes thoroughly and peel. Make a coating: Mix polenta with yogurt and rosemary. Cover potatoes with the coating and bake for 30 minutes at 400 degrees F. makes 4 servings.

Per serving: 89 calories, sodium 12 mg, potassium 233 mg, sugars 1.5 g

34. Sweet potato, beans and avocado salad

Benefits: This recipe is the best option if you're looking for something packed with protein and fiber.

Ingredients:

- 1 medium sweet potato
- 1 ripe avocado
- 1can black beans
- 1 tbsp. lemon juice
- coriander
- parsley

How to prepare: Peel sweet potato and cut into cubes. Bake until tender. Meanwhile combine mashed avocado, beans, coriander and parsley. Add sweet potato, mix well. Drizzle with lemon juice and serve slightly warm. Makes 3 servings.

Per serving: 172 calories, sodium 19 mg, potassium 512 mg, sugars 3 g

35. Spicy carrot rice

Benefits: This low fat recipe is the best option to impress your relatives and friends. Cashews add a whole lot of benefits to this recipe: they are packed with copper, manganese, magnesium, phosphorus, iron, selenium, and vitamin B6.

Ingredients:

- 100 g brown rice or black rice
- 2 small carrots
- 1 medium red onion
- 1 medium tomato
- 30 g cashews
- cinnamon
- coriander

How to prepare: Chop the onion, tomato, shred the carrots, add cinnamon and coriander and fry for 15 minutes on low heat. Meanwhile cook your rice as stated on the packaging. Combine vegetable sauce, rice and crumbled cashews. Serve immediately. Makes 4 servings.

Per serving: 160 calories, sodium 22 mg, potassium 302 mg, sugars 3 g

36. Pineapple, corn and curry quinoa

Benefits: Pineapple is a great source of potassium, copper, manganese, calcium, magnesium, vitamin C, beta carotene, thiamin, B6, and folate.

Ingredients:

- 80 g quinoa
- 100 g pineapple
- 1 can sweet corn
- curry powder

How to prepare: Cook the quinoa according to the packaging. Chop the pineapple, add corn and curry powder. Combine your mixture with cooked quinoa and serve cold. Makes 3 servings.

Per serving: 156 calories, sodium 2 mg, potassium 306 mg, sugars 5 g

37. Baked zucchini with mushrooms and pine nuts

Benefits: Pine nuts contain nutrients that help boost energy levels and are also a good source of magnesium.

Ingredients:

- 1 medium zucchini
- 100 g mushrooms
- 40 g pine nuts
- 2 tbsp. olive oil
- 1 tbsp. garlic powder

How to prepare: Cut zucchini into rings, dice the onions, add garlic powder, and pine nuts. Drizzle with olive oil and bake for 30 minutes at 375 degrees F. Makes 3 servings.

Per serving: 197 calories, sodium 9 mg, potassium 388 mg, sugars 3 g

38. Sweet potato pudding with mixed nuts

Benefits: Sweet potato is high in protein and has an awesome taste that goes well in both sweet and savory recipes. Nuts are packed with potassium and magnesium, essential minerals to lower your high blood pressure.

Ingredients:

- 1 medium sweet potato
- 1 cup coconut milk or low fat milk
- 1 tbsp. honey
- 50 g mixed nuts (walnuts, pistachios, hazelnuts etc.)

How to prepare: Boil sweet potato and put in a blender, pour in coconut milk, and honey. Add mixed nuts and blend well. Distribute the mixture between 3 separate cups and leave in a freezer overnight.

Per serving: 208 calories, sodium 162 mg, potassium 416 mg, sugars 12 g

39. Spring onion buckwheat flat cakes

Benefits: Spring onion is high in Vitamin C, Vitamin B2, thiamine, Vitamin A, Vitamin K, copper, phosphorous, magnesium, potassium, chromium, manganese and fiber. Spring onions can boost your immune system and help prevent multiple illnesses like heart disease.

Ingredients:

- 30 g spring onion
- 50 g buckwheat flour
- 1 egg
- coriander
- parsley
- dill

How to prepare: Finely chop the spring onion, combine with coriander, parsley and dill. Mix 1 egg with the buckwheat flour and onion. Fry on both sides. Makes 4 small flat cakes.

Per serving: 60 calories, sodium 18 mg, potassium 108 mg, sugars 0.6 g

40. Risotto with cherries, cranberries and coconut

Benefits: Cherries contain fiber, vitamin C, carotenoids, and help prevent cancer or even from a having a stroke. They are also very good for weight loss. Cranberries are a very good source of vitamin C, dietary fiber, manganese, vitamin E, vitamin K, copper, and pantothenic acid.

Ingredients:

- 100 g rice
- 100 ml low fat milk or coconut milk
- 50 g cherries
- 30 g candied cranberries
- shredded coconut (to taste)
- almond flakes (optional)
- 2 tbsp. honey

How to prepare: Bring milk to a boil and add rice while stirring constantly. Cook the rice on low heat until the mixture resembles rice porridge. Add the berries and honey. Mix well. Sprinkle with shredded coconut and almond flakes. Makes 3 servings.

Per serving: 198 calories, sodium 20 mg, potassium 115 mg, sugars 14 g

41. Apples and celery soup

Benefits: Celery is very rich in vitamin K, folate, vitamin A, potassium, vitamin C, and dietary fiber. This light soup is low in calories and fat.

Ingredients:

- 100 g celery
- 2 medium apples
- 100 ml vegetable stock
- 1 medium onion
- 2 tbsp. olive oil

How to prepare: Heat 2 tbsp. olive oil in a medium saucepan, add finely chopped onion and fry until golden brown. Add shredded apple and celery. Pour in vegetable stock and 50 ml water. Cook on low heat for 30 minutes. Makes 3 servings.

Per serving: 163 calories, sodium 29 mg, potassium 270 mg, sugars 15 g

42. Beetroot carrot soup

Benefits: Beetroots can improve digestion and lower blood pressure. This soup is packed with delicious vegetables that go amazingly well together and are essential for weight loss.

Ingredients:

- 1 medium beetroot
- 2 medium carrots
- 1 giant potato
- 100 ml vegetable stock
- 1 small zucchini
- 1 medium tomato

Ingredients: Wash thoroughly and peel beetroot, carrots, zucchini and potatoes. Add chopped tomatoes and cover with vegetable stock and 200 ml water. Bring to a boil and simmer for 40 minutes on low heat. Serve warm. Makes 4 servings.

Per serving:74 calories, sodium 61 mg, potassium 556 mg, sugars 7 g

43. Buckwheat shakshuka

Benefits: Buckwheat and tomato sauce go incredibly well together and create a unique flavor.

Ingredients:

- 150 g tomato puree
- 2 small eggs
- 50 g buckwheat
- 1 medium red onion
- parsley
- dill
- cumin
- paprika

How to prepare: Roughly chop the onion and fry in olive oil until golden brown, add tomato puree and leave to simmer on low heat for 10 minutes, gradually adding your spices. Break 2 eggs and drop into the sauce pan and don't stir. Cover with a lid and leave on the stove until eggs are ready. Meanwhile cook your buckwheat in slightly salted water according to the packaging. Serve two dishes alongside. Makes 2 servings.

Per serving:103 calories, sodium 75 mg, potassium 459 mg, sugars 6 g

44. Summer vegetables bake

Benefits: Bell peppers as well as cherry tomatoes are packed with healthy nutrients, they have anti-cancer and blood pressure lowering properties.

Ingredients:

- 100 g cherry tomatoes
- 100 g yellow cherry tomatoes
- 2 medium red onions
- 1 small yellow bell pepper

How to prepare: Cut onions into large pieces, chop the pepper and half cherry tomatoes. Combine together and drizzle with olive oil. Bake for 30 minutes at 400 degrees F. Makes 3 servings.

Per serving: 49 calories, sodium 7 mg, potassium 317 mg, sugars 6 g

45. Spinach broccoli lentils

Benefits: Combining the two ultimate greens (broccoli and spinach) with lentils is surely a good choice. Lentils are an excellent source of molybdenum, folate, dietary fiber, copper, phosphorus, manganese, iron, protein, vitamin B1, pantothenic acid, zinc, potassium and vitamin B6.

Ingredients:

- 100 g broccoli
- fresh spinach leaves
- 50 g red lentils
- 30 g low fat cheese

How to prepare: Chop spinach leaves, broccoli, add lentils. Put mixture into a saucepan, cover with water. Cook on low heat until all the liquid is incorporated and lentils are ready. Sprinkle with grated low fat cheese. Makes 2 servings.

Per serving: 132 calories, sodium 114 mg, potassium 435 mg, sugars 1 g

46. Pistachios and avocado pesto

Benefits: Pistachios contain nutrients such as carbohydrates, proteins, fats, dietary fiber, phosphorus, potassium, thiamine, vitamin B-6, beta-carotene, calcium, iron, magnesium etc. This pesto can surely be called best healthy protein source.

Ingredients:

- 1 ripe avocado
- 30 g basil leaves
- 40 g pistachios
- 2 tbsp. olive oil

How to prepare: Blend all the ingredients together. Serve alongside mashed potatoes or on toast.

Total (300 g): 870 calories, sodium 277 mg, potassium 1477 mg, sugars 4 g

47. Summer fruit salad

Benefits: Apples, melons, blueberries and kiwis are all amazing sources of potassium and other essential healthy nutrients.

Ingredients:

- 3 medium apples
- 100 g blueberries
- 2 ripe kiwis
- 150 g melon

How to prepare: Chop all the ingredients and mix together. Makes 5 servings.

Per serving: 97 calories, sodium 7 mg, potassium 307 mg, sugars 18 g

48. Buckwheat and lentils granola

Benefits: Instead of using sugar packed granola from your local store prepare this simple healthy breakfast granola by yourself. It's rich in flavor though is so much more beneficial to your health than junk food.

Ingredients:

- 50 g buckwheat
- 50 g red lentils
- 30 g shredded coconut
- 100 g mixed nuts
- 200 ml low fat milk (or almond milk)

How to prepare: Cook the buckwheat and lentils according to the packaging. Mix them together and spread on a parchment paper in an even layer. Bake for 30 minutes at 400 degrees F. Add nuts and coconut. Pour in milk and serve. Makes 4 servings.

Per serving: 246 calories, sodium 101 mg, potassium 359 mg, sugars 5 g

ADDITIONAL TITLES FROM THIS AUTHOR

70 Effective Meal Recipes to Prevent and Solve Being Overweight: Burn Fat Fast by Using Proper Dieting and Smart Nutrition

By

Joe Correa CSN

48 Acne Solving Meal Recipes: The Fast and Natural Path to Fixing Your Acne Problems in Less Than 10 Days!

By

Joe Correa CSN

41 Alzheimer's Preventing Meal Recipes: Reduce or Eliminate Your Alzheimer's Condition in 30 Days or Less!

By

Joe Correa CSN

70 Effective Breast Cancer Meal Recipes: Prevent and Fight Breast Cancer with Smart Nutrition and Powerful Foods

By

Joe Correa CSN

Made in the USA
Monee, IL
28 January 2024

52531192R00066